Modern Dietetics at a Glance

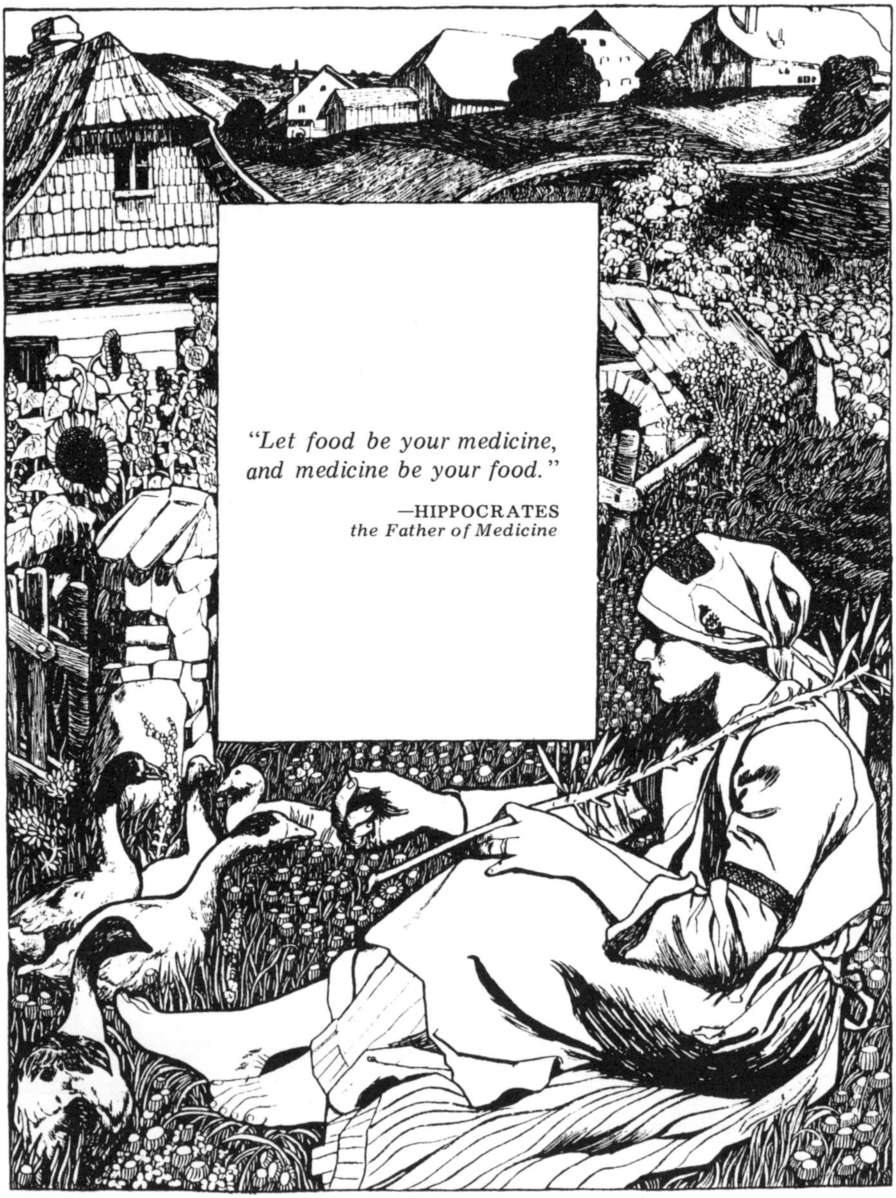

"Let food be your medicine, and medicine be your food."

—HIPPOCRATES
the Father of Medicine

Modern Dietetics at a Glance

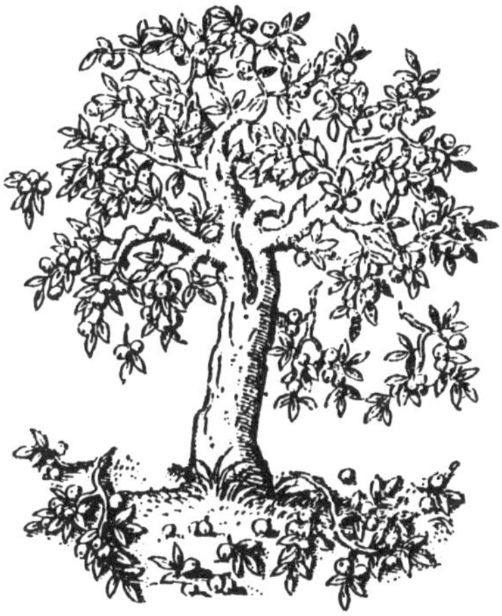

by

EDMOND BORDEAUX SZEKELY

MCMXCVII
INTERNATIONAL BIOGENIC SOCIETY

SOME BOOKS BY EDMOND BORDEAUX SZEKELY

THE ESSENE WAY—BIOGENIC LIVING
THE ESSENE GOSPEL OF PEACE, BOOK ONE
BOOK TWO, THE UNKNOWN BOOKS OF THE ESSENES
BOOK THREE, LOST SCROLLS OF THE ESSENE BROTHERHOOD
BOOK FOUR, THE TEACHINGS OF THE ELECT
THE DISCOVERY OF THE ESSENE GOSPEL: The Essenes & the Vatican
SEARCH FOR THE AGELESS, in Three Volumes
THE ESSENE BOOK OF CREATION
THE ESSENE JESUS
THE ESSENE BOOK OF ASHA
THE ZEND AVESTA OF ZARATHUSTRA
ARCHEOSOPHY, A NEW SCIENCE
THE ESSENE ORIGINS OF CHRISTIANITY
TEACHINGS OF THE ESSENES FROM ENOCH TO THE DEAD SEA SCROLLS
THE ESSENES, BY JOSEPHUS AND HIS CONTEMPORARIES
THE ESSENE TEACHINGS OF ZARATHUSTRA
THE ESSENE SCIENCE OF LIFE
THE ESSENE CODE OF LIFE
THE ESSENE SCIENCE OF FASTING AND THE ART OF SOBRIETY
ESSENE COMMUNIONS WITH THE INFINITE
THE FIRST ESSENE
THE BIOGENIC REVOLUTION
THE ORIGIN OF LIFE
THE COSMOTHERAPY OF THE ESSENES
THE LIVING BUDDHA
SIDDARTHA, THE PILGRIM
PILGRIM OF THE HIMALAYAS
MAN IN THE COSMIC OCEAN
TOWARD THE CONQUEST OF THE INNER COSMOS
FATHER, GIVE US ANOTHER CHANCE
THE ECOLOGICAL HEALTH GARDEN, THE BOOK OF SURVIVAL
THE TENDER TOUCH: BIOGENIC FULFILLMENT
THE DIALECTICAL METHOD OF THINKING
THE EVOLUTION OF HUMAN THOUGHT
THE SOUL OF ANCIENT MEXICO
ANCIENT AMERICA: PARADISE LOST
MESSENGERS FROM ANCIENT CIVILIZATIONS
SEXUAL HARMONY: THE NEW EUGENICS
LUDWIG VAN BEETHOVEN, PROMETHEUS OF THE MODERN WORLD
THE FIERY CHARIOTS
CREATIVE WORK: KARMA YOGA
THE ART OF STUDY: THE SORBONNE METHOD
COSMOS, MAN AND SOCIETY
THE BOOK OF LIVING FOODS
SCIENTIFIC VEGETARIANISM
THE CONQUEST OF DEATH
TREASURY OF RAW FOODS

Book Design by Golondrina Graphics

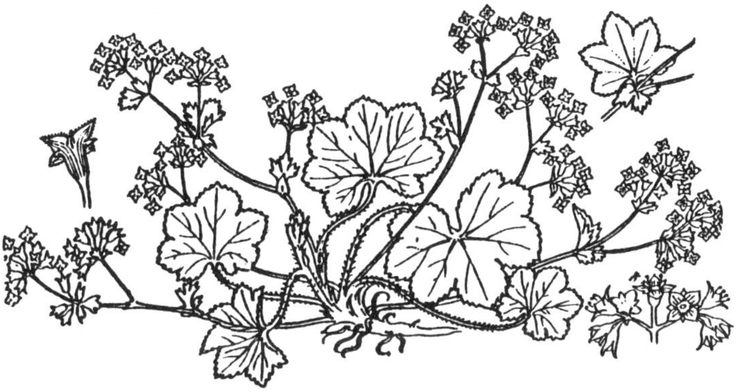

PREFACE

This present edition of *Modern Dietetics at a Glance* takes us back to 1938, when Dr. Edmond Bordeaux Szekely first wrote *Medicine Tomorrow*, a large book of 400 pages published in England. Many, many years later, he took the most important parts of *Medicine Tomorrow* and published them with the title *Cosmos, Man and Society.* This book is still available from the International Biogenic Society. He liked that title so much it apparently didn't bother him that some people would confuse this new book with another *Cosmos, Man and Society*, this one written in the early 30's, also published in England and containing 847 pages. Both this original *Cosmos, Man and Society* and *Medicine Tomorrow* are now long out of print, but before he died, Dr. Szekely chose the most important parts of the original *Cosmos, Man and Society* to appear as the following books, all available from the I.B.S.: *The Origin of Life, Healing Waters, Treasury of Raw Foods, The Evolution of Human Thought,* and *The Conquest of Death.*

So, while *Modern Dietetics at a Glance* may not be exactly "modern" anymore, it is still a very valuable collection of information from one who was truly a Renaissance man of this century, and perhaps the next. I am happy to reprint these tables and charts from the original 400-page *Medicine Tomorrow* in the hope that the information will be of help to those who are truly seeking better health and vitality through the use of natural, raw, wholesome and unprocessed foods.

the 28th of November, 1997.

—Norma Nilsson Bordeaux Szekely

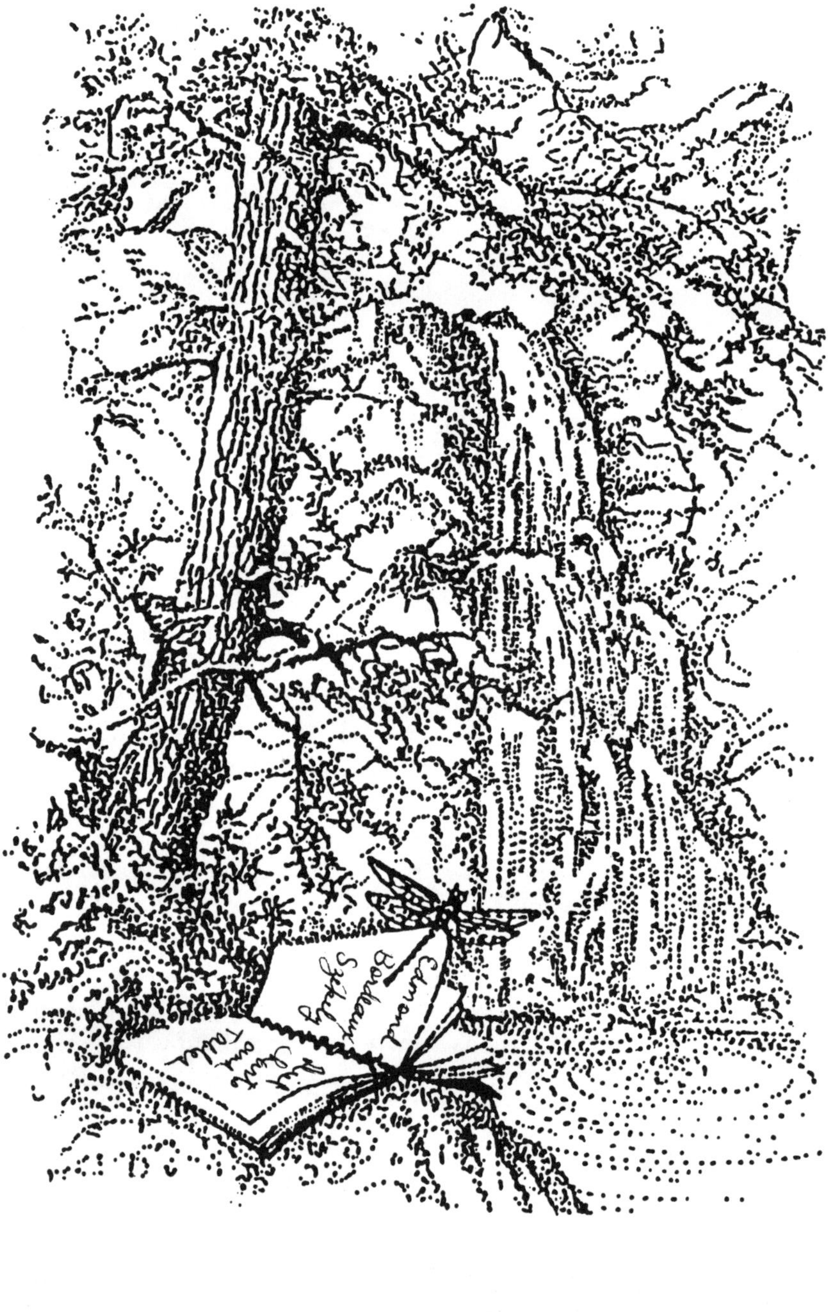
Edmond
Bordeaux
Szekely

These Charts Represent the Optimal Dietetic
Utilization of Vitamins, Calories,
Mineral Matter and other Physiochemical Properties
Accumulated in the Following Health-Giving
Foods of the Vegetable Kingdom

REFERENCE No.	NAMES OF PARTS OF BODY AND OF FOODS	IMPONDERABLE COSMOVITAL FORCES			AVERAGE CHEMICAL COMPOSITION PER CENT					COMPOSITION OF MINERAL MATTER IN 1,000 PARTS OF WATER FREE SUBSTANCE										
										ACID BINDING ELEMENTS					ACID FORMING ELEMENTS					
		PREDOMINANT RADIATIONS	PREDOMINANT VITAMINS	CALORIES Per 100 Grams	WATER	PROTEIN	FAT	CARBOHYDRATES (SUGAR, STARCH)	MINERAL MATTER	POTASSIUM K_2O	SODIUM Na_2O	CALCIUM CaO	MAGNESIUM MgO	IRON Fe_2O_3	PHOSPHORUS P_2O_5	SULPHUR SO_3	SILICON SiO_2	CHLORINE	FLUORINE	TOTAL
					CONSTITUTION OF THE HUMAN BODY AND ITS PARTS															
	HUMAN BODY, WHOLE .	HR	ABCDE	—	60.00	19.00	15.00	1.00	5.00	3.30	3.00	70.50	2.15	0.70	32.15	4.10	1.00	7.00	1.10	125.00
	RED BLOOD CORPUSCLES	"	"	—	68.78	30.20	—	—	1.02	13.81	5.87	0.55	0.30	5.00	3.50	0.28	0.01	5.68	—	35.00
	BLOOD PLASMA . .	"	"	—	90.00	9.00	—	0.15	0.85	3.30	36.75	3.20	2.35	—	1.75	1.45	0.22	36.20	—	85.22
	BLOOD SERUM . .	"	"	—	90.75	8.24	—	0.15	0.86	3.60	41.80	3.50	2.45	—	1.60	1.55	0.22	40.00	—	94.72
	LYMPH	"	"	—	94.82	4.00	0.40	0.05	0.73	3.93	57.88	1.17	0.31	0.06	1.32	—	0.50	54.75	—	119.92
	LUNGS	"	"	—	79.25	15.20	3.65	—	1.90	1.24	24.70	1.80	3.04	0.30	46.07	1.32	0.36	6.17	—	85.00
	BRAIN	"	"	—	81.10	8.50	9.30	—	1.10	19.50	6.80	0.40	0.70	0.16	27.30	0.42	0.07	4.35	—	59.70
	LIVER	"	"	—	71.55	20.00	3.65	3.25	1.55	13.90	7.90	1.97	0.11	1.44	27.30	0.50	0.14	1.26	—	54.52
	SPLEEN	"	"	—	76.14	17.10	4.20	1.00	1.56	6.12	28.26	4.77	0.30	4.64	17.26	1.55	0.11	0.35	—	63.36
	BILE	"	"	—	89.00	—	—	—	0.85	2.88	30.35	0.85	0.32	0.14	6.27	3.83	0.21	15.06	—	59.91
	BONES, FRESH . .	"	"	—	Water	and fat	-free su	bstance		—	—	240.00	8.00	10.00	345.00	—	—	12.00	15.00	630.00
	MUSCLE TISSUE, FRESH .	"	"	—	75.50	18.70	3.70	1.00	1.10	18.00	2.80	0.40	1.80	0.20	22.00	0.60	0.40	2.80	—	49.00
	HUMAN MILK . . .	"	"	66	87.75	1.60	3.95	6.25	0.45	11.73	3.16	5.80	0.75	0.07	7.84	0.33	0.07	6.38	—	36.13
	CATEGORY I	CR	BE		50% OF THE DAILY RATION — RAW JUICY FRUITS — STRONGLY ELIMINATIVE FOODS															
	GROUP A																			
1	APPLE	CR	BE	61	85.60	0.40	0.50	13.00	0.50	11.78	8.61	1.35	2.89	0.46	4.52	2.01	1.42	—	—	33.04
2	PEAR.	"	"	63	84.40	0.60	0.50	14.10	0.40	14.00	2.17	2.05	1.52	0.25	3.90	1.45	0.38	—	—	25.72
3	PEACH	"	"	65	89.32	0.70	0.10	9.40	0.48	20.90	3.00	4.60	1.35	0.50	6.05	3.50	—	0.80	—	40.70
4	APRICOT	"	"	61	84.70	1.42	—	13.34	0.54	19.68	3.76	1.08	1.22	0.26	3.76	0.92	2.80	0.20	—	33.58
5	PLUM	"	"	76	78.40	1.00	—	20.00	0.60	16.45	0.15	2.78	1.53	0.90	4.17	1.03	0.68	—	—	27.69
6	PRUNE, FRESH . .	"	"	40	82.00	0.80	—	16.50	0.70	18.28	3.41	4.34	1.36	0.94	6.03	1.21	1.19	0.15	—	36.91
7	NECTARINE . . .	"	"	39	82.90	0.60	—	15.90	0.60	—	—	—	—	—	—	—	—	—	—	—

	GROUP B																			
	STRAWBERRY	SR	BE	44	89.90	1.00	0.60	7.70	0.80	13.72	18.53	9.23	—	3.73	7.97	2.05	7.83	1.10	—	64.16
9	RASPBERRY, BLACK	,,	,,	62	84.10	1.70	1.00	12.60	0.60	—	—	—	—	—	—	—	—	—	—	—
10	RASPBERRY, RED	,,	,,	62	88.70	1.00	—	9.70	0.60	16.50	1.90	3.15	1.75	0.05	4.50	11.50	—	2.90	—	42.25
11	HUCKLEBERRY	,,	,,	55	81.00	0.80	0.60	16.60	1.00	26.44	3.00	3.70	2.82	0.50	8.05	1.44	0.42	—	—	46.37
12	CURRANT, RED	CR	,,	61	87.95	0.30	—	11.30	0.45	12.10	0.04	1.46	0.95	0.03	2.17	7.95	—	0.35	—	25.05
13	CURRANT, WHITE	,,	,,	61	85.56	0.40	—	13.60	0.44	16.90	0.16	0.29	0.45	0.05	1.40	3.95	—	0.30	—	23.50
14	CURRANT, BLACK	,,	,,	61	79.79	1.00	—	18.70	0.51	13.70	0.13	0.60	0.75	0.04	2.27	4.73	—	0.08	—	22.30
15	BLACKBERRY	SR	,,	42	86.35	1.30	1.00	10.90	0.45	17.90	0.60	7.95	4.75	0.05	6.20	0.90	—	1.80	—	40.15
16	GOOSEBERRY	CR	,,	55	90.70	0.50	—	8.40	0.40	11.22	2.87	3.54	1.70	1.32	5.71	1.71	0.75	0.22	—	29.04
17	CRANBERRY	SR	,,	—	90.20	0.40	0.60	8.40	0.40	9.00	0.03	10.15	0.90	0.04	1.60	14.20	—	0.03	—	35.95
18	MULBERRY	CR	,,	38	84.70	0.40	—	14.30	0.60	—	—	—	—	—	—	—	—	—	—	—
19	MEDLAR	,,	,,	103	82.10	0.50	0.30	16.50	0.60	—	—	—	—	—	—	—	—	—	—	—
20	MIRABELLE	,,	,,	32	85.34	0.60	—	13.60	0.46	13.50	1.80	1.40	1.20	0.35	4.80	1.85	—	0.15	—	24.25
21	RHUBARB (JUICE)	SR	,,	18	94.40	0.60	0.70	3.60	0.70	74.50	6.45	12.55	—	1.84	18.41	2.34	3.46	6.81	—	126.36
22	GRAPE	CR	,,	40	78.20	1.30	1.25	18.60	0.65	18.75	0.40	2.70	1.25	0.45	4.00	1.50	0.60	0.35	—	30.00
23	CHERRY	,,	,,	77	80.80	1.00	0.80	16.70	0.70	17.94	0.76	2.60	1.90	0.70	5.54	1.76	3.11	0.48	—	34.59
24	POMEGRANATE	,,	,,	7	79.50	1.50	1.60	16.80	0.60	8.00	12.25	1.65	0.90	0.06	2.50	0.20	—	0.34	—	25.50
25	FIG, FRESH (BLACK)	,,	,,	81	79.00	1.50	0.20	18.70	0.60	—	—	—	—	—	—	—	—	—	—	—
26	WATERMELON	SR	,,	32	92.30	0.50	0.20	6.70	0.30	18.00	3.75	4.00	2.10	1.75	5.60	2.10	1.60	1.10	—	40.00
27	MUSKMELON	,,	,,	30	91.60	0.60	—	7.20	0.60	—	—	—	—	—	—	—	—	—	—	—
	GROUP C																			
28	LEMON	CR	,,	44	89.30	1.00	0.70	8.50	0.50	22.54	0.84	12.75	2.09	0.20	5.25	1.25	0.31	0.18	—	45.41
29	LIME	,,	,,	44	97.61	0.83	—	0.58	0.98	28.38	—	5.17	1.56	—	5.70	2.24	—	2.65	—	45.70
30	ORANGE	,,	,,	51	86.90	0.80	0.20	11.60	0.50	18.62	0.95	8.65	2.03	0.38	4.70	2.00	0.25	0.29	—	37.87
31	GRAPEFRUIT	,,	,,	48	91.68	0.56	—	7.37	0.39	13.20	—	2.20	1.20	0.38	3.32	1.00	—	0.40	—	21.70
32	MANGO	,,	,,	80	88.60	0.60	0.40	9.90	0.50	18.95	—	2.55	0.64	—	2.60	1.47	—	1.55	—	27.76
33	PAPAYA	,,	,,	4	88.59	0.50	0.05	10.30	0.56	—	—	—	—	—	—	—	—	—	—	—
34	PERSIMMON	,,	,,	—	67.90	0.80	0.70	29.70	0.90	—	—	—	—	—	—	—	—	—	—	—
35	PINEAPPLE	SR	,,	159	89.30	0.40	0.30	9.70	0.30	12.55	2.20	3.10	2.10	0.40	1.40	4.15	—	2.70	—	28.60
36	CUSTARD APPLE (CHERIMOYA)	CR	,,	—	89.80	—	—	9.16	1.04	18.40	—	0.81	0.25	—	2.43	1.67	—	2.74	—	26.30
37	CACTUS FRUIT	,,	,,	—	82.90	1.40	1.30	11.70	2.70	—	—	—	—	—	—	—	—	—	—	—
38	CACTUS LEAVES	,,	,,	—	94.66	0.70	0.09	3.30	1.23	—	—	—	—	—	—	—	—	—	—	—
39	GUAVA	,,	,,	43	89.50	1.30	0.70	8.00	0.50	15.47	—	0.75	0.48	—	2.44	1.05	0.30	1.55	—	22.04
40	GUAVA, STRAWBERRY	,,	,,	—	89.47	0.76	0.95	8.05	0.77	—	—	—	—	—	—	—	—	—	—	—
41	JUJUBE	,,	,,	—	75.96	1.44	0.21	21.66	0.73	—	—	—	—	—	—	—	—	—	—	—
42	DURIAN	,,	,,	—	70.76	2.30	—	23.70	1.24	—	—	—	—	—	—	—	—	—	—	—
43	SAPODILLA	,,	,,	—	77.58	0.87	0.55	20.00	1.00	—	—	—	—	—	—	—	—	—	—	—
44	SAPOTE, WHITE	,,	,,	—	76.36	0.87	0.55	21.75	0.47	—	—	—	—	—	—	—	—	—	—	—
45	STAR APPLE	,,	,,	—	91.57	2.35	1.38	4.40	0.40	—	—	—	—	—	—	—	—	—	—	—
46	LITCHI, FRESH	,,	,,	43	82.81	1.15	0.20	15.30	0.54	—	—	—	—	—	—	—	—	—	—	—
47	LITCHI, DRIED	,,	,,	—	16.40	2.90	0.80	78.00	1.90	—	—	—	—	—	—	—	—	—	—	—
48	TAMARIND	,,	,,	132	65.65	1.36	—	31.43	1.56	—	—	—	—	—	—	—	—	—	—	—

ABBREVIATIONS: C=Cosmic S=Solar T=Terrestrial H=Human A=Animal R=Radiations

REFERENCE No.	NAMES OF PARTS OF BODY AND OF FOODS	IMPONDERABLE COSMOVITAL FORCES			AVERAGE CHEMICAL COMPOSITION PER CENT					COMPOSITION OF MINERAL MATTER IN 1,000 PARTS OF WATER FREE SUBSTANCE										
										ACID BINDING ELEMENTS					ACID FORMING ELEMENTS					
		PREDOMINANT RADIATIONS	PREDOMINANT VITAMINS	CALORIES Per 100 Grams	WATER	PROTEIN	FAT	CARBOHYDRATES (SUGAR, STARCH)	MINERAL MATTER	POTASSIUM K_2O	SODIUM Na_2O	CALCIUM CaO	MAGNESIUM MgO	IRON Fe_2O_3	PHOSPHORUS P_2O_5	SULPHUR SO_3	SILICON SiO_2	CHLORINE	FLUORINE	TOTAL
	CATEGORY II	TR-SR	ABCE		35% OF THE DAILY RATION — RAW VEGETABLES — ELIMINATIVE FOODS															
	GROUP A																			
49	TOMATO	SR	ABCE	24	94.10	0.90	0.20	3.75	1.05	82.50	32.90	11.35	13.55	1.00	10.75	5.00	1.75	18.00	—	176.80
50	CUCUMBER	,,	,,	16	95.96	1.20	0.10	2.30	0.44	41.20	18.00	7.30	4.15	1.40	20.20	6.90	8.00	6.60	—	105.75
	GROUP B																			
51	TURNIP	TR	,,	36	83.82	3.50	0.10	11.30	1.28	59.10	7.10	14.24	4.66	0.75	18.27	12.10	1.40	8.30	—	125.92
52	TURNIP LEAF	SR	,,	47	—	—	—	—	—	22.63	8.16	27.39	2.78	1.29	3.71	4.38	—	—	—	70.34
53	RADISH (LARGE)	TR	,,	24	89.53	1.90	0.10	7.40	1.07	18.00	3.05	6.60	2.85	1.00	33.70	6.35	6.75	4.00	—	82.30
54	RADISH (SMALL)	,,	,,	24	94.11	1.20	0.15	3.80	0.74	35.10	23.15	16.30	3.35	3.00	12.00	7.15	1.00	10.00	—	111.05
55	PARSNIP	,,	,,	61	83.00	1.60	0.50	13.50	1.40	33.80	0.32	4.80	2.50	0.25	10.25	8.00	9.60	10.40	—	79.92
56	BEETROOT	,,	,,	32	87.50	1.60	0.10	9.70	1.10	38.70	9.00	5.45	2.73	0.26	8.27	6.15	7.90	9.00	—	87.46
57	SUGAR BEET	,,	,,	31	82.40	1.00	0.10	15.80	0.70	20.15	3.35	2.30	3.00	0.45	4.60	1.60	—	1.85	—	37.30
58	SUGAR BEET LEAF	SR	,,	28	88.75	1.91	0.03	8.64	0.70	23.40	11.00	15.60	7.35	0.40	3.25	2.60	—	—	—	63.60
59	BEETROOT, RED	TR	,,	44	88.00	1.20	0.20	10.10	0.50	8.45	21.60	2.50	0.10	1.00	2.55	6.50	2.00	2.95	—	41.65
60	KOHLRABI	SR	,,	42	85.53	4.90	0.20	8.20	1.17	29.30	5.40	9.15	5.65	2.50	1.70	7.35	2.05	4.10	—	67.20
61	CARROT	TR	,,	47	87.50	1.00	0.20	9.40	0.90	25.46	14.63	7.80	3.04	0.70	8.83	4.45	1.66	3.18	—	69.75
62	OXALIS (SORREL)	,,	,,	32	93.12	1.70	0.30	3.90	0.98	56.05	0.85	7.00	8.70	9.85	21.35	13.30	—	8.70	—	125.80
63	ARTICHOKE	,,	,,	75	80.26	1.80	0.14	16.70	1.10	25.32	5.38	1.75	1.55	2.00	7.40	2.60	5.30	2.06	—	53.36
64	JERUSALEM ARTICHOKE	,,	,,	78	80.35	1.50	0.10	17.00	1.05	26.20	5.80	1.80	1.60	2.15	7.65	2.70	—	2.10	—	50.00

	GROUP C																			
65	LETTUCE	SR	..	19	95.07	1.40	0.30	2.20	1.03	67.94	13.55	26.56	11.20	9.40	16.62	6.87	14.64	13.82	—	180.60
66	LETTUCE, ROMAINE	..	..	19	92.50	1.54	0.43	4.20	1.33	44.90	62.70	21.10	7.60	2.30	19.40	6.90	5.30	7.40	—	177.60
67	LETTUCE, LAMBS'	..	..	20	93.41	2.70	0.40	2.70	0.79	53.00	11.20	7.20	2.60	0.45	10.20	5.80	24.00	5.70	—	120.15
68	BRUSSELS SPROUTS	SR	..	58	88.03	3.50	0.30	6.80	1.37	31.40	0.35	2.40	2.35	0.60	20.25	35.30	—	2.75	—	95.40
69	CABBAGE	..	..	48	91.87	1.90	0.20	4.80	1.23	45.38	11.68	21.65	4.90	0.86	11.07	17.10	1.10	10.45	—	124.19
70	CABBAGE, SAVOY	..	..	32	88.36	3.30	0.70	6.00	1.64	34.80	12.95	27.17	8.13	2.16	18.63	10.41	6.07	10.03	—	130.35
71	CABBAGE, RED.	..	..	25	91.34	1.83	0.20	5.86	0.77	17.00	9.33	21.48	3.41	0.08	3.00	9.58	0.38	10.51	—	74.77
72	CAULIFLOWER	..	..	33	91.82	2.50	0.30	4.55	0.83	40.46	5.38	5.10	3.37	0.91	18.42	11.86	3.37	3.10	—	91.97
73	OKRA	..	..	—	90.20	1.60	0.20	7.40	0.60	8.80	12.00	21.00	3.30	0.01	9.00	7.10	—	—	—	61.21
74	DANDELION	..	..	—	87.15	2.80	0.70	7.45	1.90	50.95	13.63	26.20	11.00	1.10	10.22	2.88	9.17	3.47	—	128.52
75	LEEK BULB	..	..	42	88.26	2.80	0.30	6.50	1.24	30.70	14.15	10.40	2.90	7.60	16.70	7.40	7.40	3.10	—	100.35
76	LEEK LEAF	..	..	50	92.21	1.50	0.30	5.10	0.69	33.25	5.55	17.70	3.60	0.50	6.25	3.35	—	5.50	—	75.70
77	ASPARAGUS	..	..	23	94.81	1.80	0.25	2.60	0.54	20.94	14.77	9.33	3.72	2.94	16.07	5.36	9.50	5.10	—	87.69
78	SWISS CHARD	..	..	—	92.50	1.54	0.43	4.20	1.33	44.90	62.70	21.70	7.60	2.30	19.40	6.90	5.30	7.40	—	178.20
	GROUP D																			
79	CELERY	..	..	18	94.50	1.10	0.10	3.30	1.00	48.60	65.25	14.70	6.75	1.60	14.50	6.50	4.30	17.80	—	180.00
80	CELERY ROOT	TR	..	18	85.46	1.50	0.40	11.80	0.84	22.70	—	6.90	3.05	0.75	6.75	2.95	2.10	8.45	—	53.65
81	SPINACH	SR	..	32	89.36	3.50	0.60	4.44	2.10	29.90	63.90	21.50	11.50	6.05	18.05	12.45	8.10	11.30	—	182.75
82	WATERCRESS	..	..	27	95.24	1.90	0.10	1.30	1.46	44.75	17.25	35.00	8.60	0.35	22.40	53.90	—	7.75	—	190.00
83	CHICKORY ROOT	TR	..	20	79.97	0.80	0.20	18.30	0.73	13.20	5.05	2.40	1.60	0.85	4.30	2.70	—	2.75	—	32.85
84	GREEN PEPPER	SR	..	—	93.20	1.10	0.10	4.60	1.00	—	—	—	—	—	—	—	—	—	—	—
85	SALSIFY	TR	..	75	87.40	4.30	0.30	6.80	1.20	—	—	—	—	—	—	—	—	—	—	—
86	SALSIFY (BLACK)	..	..	—	80.40	1.00	0.50	17.10	1.00	15.30	6.40	3.40	2.07	1.48	12.95	5.60	—	1.60	—	48.80
87	KALE	SR	..	56	93.42	1.90	0.10	3.00	1.58	81.50	5.35	28.10	7.30	1.30	35.50	86.00	—	10.50	—	255.55
88	RUTABAGA	..	..	—	88.90	1.30	0.20	8.50	1.10	46.30	13.60	8.80	5.20	1.70	18.10	5.30	—	1.00	—	100.00
	GROUP E																			
89	COW'S MILK, FRESH RAW	SAR	..	67	87.16	3.55	3.70	4.88	0.71	13.70	5.34	12.24	1.69	0.30	15.79	0.17	0.02	8.04	—	57.29
90	GOAT'S MILK, FRESH RAW	..	..	71	87.00	4.30	4.50	4.40	0.80	15.60	3.45	13.90	2.30	0.60	21.05	0.30	0.20	13.50	—	70.90
91	SHEEP'S MILK, FRESH RAW	..	..	107	80.80	6.50	6.90	4.90	0.90	5.03	4.65	11.70	2.15	0.17	17.70	0.20	0.10	5.70	—	47.40
92	BUTTERMILK	..	..	35	91.00	3.00	0.50	4.80	0.70	18.10	8.50	14.40	2.60	0.60	21.80	1.30	—	9.70	—	77.00
93	SKIM-MILK	..	..	35	90.50	3.40	0.30	5.10	0.70	22.60	7.10	15.20	2.20	0.60	13.40	2.40	—	10.20	—	73.70
94	WHEY	..	..	32	93.79	0.60	0.07	5.10	0.44	21.85	9.75	13.65	0.25	0.40	12.00	1.90	—	11.20	—	71.00
	GROUP F				1-5% OF THE DAILY RATION — CONDIMENTS WITH OIL AND LEMON JUICE FOR SALADS															
95	CHIVE	TR	..	—	85.75	2.80	0.50	10.00	0.95	18.05	2.28	11.27	2.90	0.80	8.12	6.66	—	2.32	—	52.40
96	ONION	..	..	49	87.60	1.60	0.30	9.90	0.60	12.10	1.55	10.65	2.55	2.20	7.25	2.65	8.10	1.35	—	48.40
97	GARLIC	..	..	142	63.70	6.80	0.10	27.90	1.50	—	—	—	—	—	—	—	—	—	—	—
98	DILL	SR	..	—	85.90	3.50	0.90	7.30	2.40	28.70	12.65	31.95	11.55	1.00	20.30	20.05	2.40	14.75	—	143.35
99	PARSLEY	..	..	70	86.45	3.70	8.70	7.45	1.70	—	—	—	—	—	—	—	—	—	—	—
100	HORSERADISH	TR	..	—	79.45	2.70	0.35	16.00	1.50	19.81	2.57	5.28	1.87	1.25	4.96	19.84	8.18	8.18	—	71.94

ABBREVIATIONS: C=Cosmic S=Solar T=Terrestrial H=Human A=Animal R=Radiations

REFERENCE No.	NAMES OF FOODS (Continued)	IMPONDERABLE COSMOVITAL FORCES: PREDOMINANT RADIATIONS	IMPONDERABLE COSMOVITAL FORCES: PREDOMINANT VITAMINS	IMPONDERABLE COSMOVITAL FORCES: CALORIES Per 100 Grams	AVERAGE CHEMICAL COMPOSITION PER CENT: WATER	PROTEIN	FAT	CARBOHYDRATES (SUGAR, STARCH)	MINERAL MATTER	COMPOSITION OF MINERAL MATTER IN 1000 PARTS OF WATER FREE SUBSTANCE — ACID BINDING ELEMENTS: POTASSIUM K_2O	SODIUM Na_2O	CALCIUM CaO	MAGNESIUM MgO	IRON Fe_2O_3	ACID FORMING ELEMENTS: PHOSPHORUS P_2O_5	SULPHUR SO_3	SILICON SiO_2	CHLORINE	FLUORINE	TOTAL
	CATEGORY III	SR	BE		10% OF THE DAILY RATION — CEREALS AND STARCHES — RECONSTRUCTIVE FOODS															
	GROUP A																			
101	BANANA	CR	,,	99	75.30	1.30	0.60	22.00	0.80	16.10	5.60	0.68	2.40	0.07	2.85	1.20	0.50	2.70	—	32.40
102	POTATO	TR	,,	95	75.67	2.08	0.15	21.00	1.10	26.56	1.33	1.15	2.18	0.48	7.47	2.89	0.83	1.55	—	44.49
103	SWEET POTATO	,,	,,	—	69.00	1.80	0.70	27.40	1.10	18.60	2.20	3.10	0.85	0.50	2.20	1.05	1.40	5.50	—	35.40
104	BREADFRUIT	CR	,,	—	82.17	1.57	0.51	14.60	1.15	17.50	2.10	6.30	0.50	0.01	5.10	3.75	—	1.50	—	36.76
	GROUP B																			
105	WHEAT, WHOLE	SR	,,	352	13.40	13.60	1.90	69.10	2.00	7.20	0.50	0.75	2.80	0.30	10.90	0.09	0.46	0.07	—	23.07
106	WHEAT, GERM OF	,,	,,	379	12.30	35.70	13.10	31.20	5.70	—	—	—	—	—	—	—	—	—	—	—
107	WHEAT, BRAN	,,	,,	323	12.95	16.60	3.50	62.10	4.85	15.15	0.33	1.65	9.35	0.38	27.80	0.13	0.50	—	—	55.29
108	WHEAT BREAD, WHOLE	,,	,,	251	35.70	8.90	1.80	52.10	1.50	4.15	4.10	1.55	1.05	0.30	4.75	0.60	—	6.80	—	23.30
109	PUMPERNICKEL BREAD	,,	,,	223	50.45	4.20	0.70	43.30	1.35	2.35	6.40	1.50	2.35	0.45	4.50	0.85	—	4.80	—	23.20
110	SWEDISH RYE CRISP	,,	,,	370	18.45	8.00	0.60	70.10	1.95	5.60	2.70	1.00	1.20	0.08	5.85	2.90	—	1.90	—	21.23
	GERMINATED WHEAT GRAIN—																			
111	WHOLE	,,	,,																	
112	CRUSHED	,,	,,																	
113	SUN-BAKED	,,	,,	352	13.40	13.60	1.90	69.10	2.00	7.20	0.50	0.75	2.80	0.30	10.90	0.09	0.46	0.07	—	23.07
114	OVEN-BAKED	,,	,,		(Average figures. Exact figures depend on proportion of water used)															
115	BOILED	,,	,,																	

	GROUP C																				
116	RYE, WHOLE	,,	,,	370	17.09	11.50	1.80	67.80	1.81	6.84	0.31	0.61	2.39	0.25	10.16	0.28	0.30	0.01	—	21.15
117	CORN, WHOLE YELLOW (MAIZE)	,,	,,	343	15.54	9.85	4.60	68.50	1.51	5.50	0.20	0.36	2.87	0.15	8.44	0.15	0.39	0.35	—	18.41
118	CORN, GREEN (MAIZE)	,,	,,	—	75.90	3.10	1.10	19.20	0.70	8.50	3.20	0.50	2.65	0.07	8.28	3.68	0.50	1.12	—	28.50
119	CORN, POPPED	,,	,,	363	5.70	10.70	5.00	77.30	1.30	—	—	—	—	—	—	—	—	—	—	—
120	RICE, WHOLE	,,	,,	350	13.87	7.85	0.88	76.50	1.00	3.60	0.67	0.59	1.78	0.22	8.60	0.10	0.40	0.02	—	15.98
121	RICE, BRAN	,,	,,	—	14.40	11.10	7.85	62.10	4.55	6.00	—	1.35	9.15	4.00	22.85	0.12	8.85	—	—	52.30
122	MILLET	,,	,,	355	15.00	9.00	3.80	70.25	1.95	4.46	0.71	0.28	3.26	0.42	13.00	—	1.60	—	—	23.73
123	OATS, WHOLE	,,	,,	410	23.58	10.40	5.20	57.80	3.02	10.40	1.35	2.25	4.25	0.40	14.30	0.80	0.40	0.35	—	34.50
124	OATS, ROLLED	,,	,,	410	7.70	16.70	7.30	66.20	2.10	6.50	1.30	1.50	2.10	0.60	7.15	1.45	0.20	0.60	—	21.40
125	OATMEAL	,,	,,	380	7.30	16.05	7.20	67.50	1.95	5.50	1.00	1.10	1.75	0.05	8.10	1.40	0.20	1.10	—	20.20
126	BUCK WHEAT	,,	,,	343	14.74	11.41	2.68	68.79	2.38	6.32	1.68	1.21	3.41	0.47	13.35	0.55	0.06	0.35	—	27.40
127	BARLEY, WHOLE	,,	,,	339	19.10	11.10	2.20	64.90	2.70	8.80	1.05	1.10	3.70	0.40	15.00	0.70	0.20	0.35	—	31.30
	GROUP D																				
128	SORGHUM	,,	,,	—	15.40	9.10	3.60	69.80	2.10	6.00	0.90	0.35	5.20	0.58	10.60	0.12	—	0.25	—	24.00
129	SAGO	,,	,,	346	12.20	9.00	0.40	78.10	0.30	—	—	—	—	—	—	—	—	—	—	—
130	TAPIOCA	TR	,,	350	11.40	0.40	0.10	88.00	0.10	—	—	—	—	—	—	—	—	—	—	—
131	TARO	,,	,,	100	73.00	1.80	0.20	23.20	1.20	—	—	—	—	—	—	—	—	—	—	—
132	YAM	,,	,,	100	73.80	1.80	0.20	23.30	0.90	—	—	—	—	—	—	—	—	—	—	—
133	CASSAVA, SWEET	,,	,,	100	67.80	1.10	0.20	30.20	0.70	—	—	—	—	—	—	—	—	—	—	—

ABBREVIATIONS: C=Cosmic S=Solar T=Terrestrial H=Human A=Animal R=Radiations

REFERENCE No.	NAMES OF FOODS (Continued)	IMPONDERABLE COSMOVITAL FORCES: PREDOMINANT RADIATIONS	PREDOMINANT VITAMINS	CALORIES Per 100 Grams	AVERAGE CHEMICAL COMPOSITION PER CENT: WATER	PROTEIN	FAT	CARBOHYDRATES (SUGAR, STARCH)	MINERAL MATTER	COMPOSITION OF MINERAL MATTER IN 1000 PARTS OF WATER FREE SUBSTANCE — ACID BINDING ELEMENTS: POTASSIUM K_2O	SODIUM Na_2O	CALCIUM CaO	MAGNESIUM MgO	IRON Fe_2O_3	ACID FORMING ELEMENTS: PHOSPHORUS P_2O_5	SULPHUR SO_3	SILICON SiO_2	CHLORINE	FLUORINE	TOTAL
	CATEGORY IV	CR-AR	ABD		5% OF THE DAILY RATION — DRIED, SWEET AND OILY FRUITS AND ANIMAL PRODUCTS—STRONGLY RECONSTRUCTIVE FOODS															
	GROUP A																			
134	RAISIN	CR	..	296	17.10	2.60	3.30	73.60	3.40	19.40	3.30	2.45	2 30	0.60	7.30	2.55	—	2.10	—	40.[illegible]0
135	PRUNE	..	..	302	24.40	2.10	—	71.20	2.30	19.15	0.80	1.40	1.75	0.80	4.20	0.80	0.90	0.10	—	29.[illegible]8
136	FIG, DRIED (SMYRNA)	..	..	276	18.80	4.30	0.30	74.20	2.40	17.10	0.90	3.30	1.68	0.66	3.85	1.20	—	0.61	—	29 30
137	FIG, DRIED (BLACK)	..	..	276	27.30	5.50	1.00	63.00	3.20	10.50	9.60	3.50	3.40	0.60	6.30	2.70	2.40	1.00	—	40.[illegible]
138	DATE	..	..	308	23.50	2.10	2.80	70.00	1.60	10.50	1.00	1.15	1.19	0.06	1.00	1.20	—	3.90	—	20.00
139	APPLE, DRIED	..	..	250	33.20	1.60	2.20	62.00	2.00	—	—	—	—	—	—	—	—	—	—	—
140	APRICOT, DRIED	..	..	225	29.40	4.70	1.00	62.50	2.40	—	—	—	—	—	—	—	—	—	—	—
141	PEAR, DRIED	..	..	252	23.40	2.80	5.40	66.00	2.40	—	—	—	—	—	—	—	—	—	—	—
142	PEACH, DRIED	..	..	254	24.25	3.15	0.45	50.00	2.15	—	—	—	—	—	—	—	—	—	—	—
143	CURRANT, DRIED (ZANTE)	..	..	180	17.20	2.40	1.70	74.20	4.50	30.00	3.15	1.60	1.85	0.30	12.40	3.10	—	1.75	—	54.15
	GROUP B																			
144	HONEY	CSAR	..	321	18.20	0.40	—	81.20	0.20	0.02	0.10	2.35	0.01	0.12	0.18	0.01	—	0.01	—	2.80
145	SUGAR CANE	SR	..	100	75.43	1.50	0.55	21.82	0.70	—	—	—	—	—	—	—	—	—	—	28.40
146	RAW SUGAR	STR	..	350	4.14	0.30	—	94.60	0.96	5.97	1.30	0.70	0.03	0.04	0.03	0.95	—	0.78	—	9.80
147	MOLASSES	SR	..	246	25.10	2.40	—	69.30	3.20	27.00	0.38	4.22	1.36	0.02	0.88	2.58	—	6.34	—	42.78

	GROUP C																			
148	ALMOND	CR	,,	639	4.90	21.40	54.40	16.80	2.50	5.23	0.38	3.04	3.95	0.23	10.10	0.96	0.04	0.06	—	23.99
149	WALNUT, ENGLISH	,,	,,	754	2.50	18.40	64.40	13.00	1.70	2.20	0.17	0.97	2.88	0.61	10.10	0.22	0.12	0.12	—	17.39
150	WALNUT, BLACK	,,	,,	731	2.50	27.60	56.30	11.70	1.90	—	—	—	—	—	—	—	—	—	—	—
151	BRAZIL NUT	,,	,,	742	8.60	17.40	65.90	5.70	3.30	6.65	0.37	6.10	2.90	0.10	13.30	4.33	—	0.85	—	34.60
152	PECAN	,,	,,	—	7.10	12.10	70.70	8.50	1.60	5.80	0.36	1.33	2.20	0.23	6.75	—	—	—	—	16.67
153	BUTTERNUT	,,	,,	—	4.50	27.90	61.29	3.40	3.00	—	—	—	—	—	—	—	—	—	—	—
154	PARADISE NUT	,,	,,	—	2.30	22.20	62.60	10.20	2.70	—	—	—	—	—	—	—	—	—	—	—
155	CANDLENUT	,,	,,	—	8.67	21.40	61.70	4.90	3.30	—	—	—	—	—	—	—	—	—	—	—
156	CHESTNUT, DRIED	,,	,,	620	5.90	10.70	7.00	74.20	2.20	11.40	0.28	1.07	1.87	0.14	5.50	3.00	0.04	0.01	—	23.31
157	WATER CHESTNUT	,,	,,	194	42.93	4.00	1.20	50.00	1.77	12.30	0.01	0.90	0.15	0.01	5.10	0.45	—	0.15	—	19.07
158	COCOANUT	,,	,,	500	14.10	5.70	50.60	27.90	1.70	9.75	1.30	1.10	1.30	0.40	4.80	0.85	—	3.20	—	22.70
159	COCOANUT, DRIED	,,	,,	600	3.50	6.30	57.40	31.50	1.30	—	—	—	—	—	—	—	—	—	—	—
160	COCOANUT MILK	,,	,,	4	92.70	0.40	1.50	4.60	0.80	—	—	—	—	—	—	—	—	—	—	—
161	PIGNOLIA, ITALIAN	,,	,,	—	6.20	33.90	48.20	7.90	3.80	—	—	—	—	—	—	—	—	—	—	—
162	PISTACHIO	,,	,,	—	4.20	22.60	54.50	15.60	3.10	—	—	—	—	—	—	—	—	—	—	—
163	HICKORY NUT	,,	,,	700	3.70	15.40	67.40	11.40	2.10	—	—	—	—	—	—	—	—	—	—	—
164	BEECH NUT	,,	,,	—	12.74	21.70	42.50	19.20	3.86	7.20	2.18	7.73	5.94	0.42	12.81	1.03	1.13	1.03	—	39.47
165	PINON	,,	,,	617	3.30	14.60	61.90	17.30	2.90	5.70	0.75	2.62	4.20	0.60	13.15		—	—	—	27.02
166	FILBERT	,,	,,	636	5.40	16.50	64.00	11.70	2.40	6.65	0.20	3.60	1.98	0.46	7.30	4.46	—	0.60	—	25.05
167	PEANUT	SR	,,	554	9.75	29.80	43.50	14.70	2.25	9.27	0.21	0.95	2.29	0.27	10.60	0.45	0.05	0.23	—	24.32
168	PEANUT BUTTER	,,	,,	930	4.90	29.30	46.50	17.10	2.20	—	—	—	—	—	—	—	—	—	—	—
169	ALMOND BUTTER	CR	,,	930	2.20	21.70	61.50	11.60	3.00	—	—	—	—	—	—	—	—	—	—	—
170	CAROB (ST. JOHN'S BREAD)	,,	,,	—	23.70	5.70	1.10	67.00	2.50	—	—	—	—	—	—	—	—	—	—	—
171	COCOA BEAN	SR	,,	490	8.80	12.00	49.30	26.40	3.50	12.96	0.82	1.95	4.00	0.02	13.95	1.25	0.55	0.30	—	35.80
172	AVOCADO	CR	,,	—	70.55	2.10	20.00	6.00	1.35	11.75	8.35	2.15	2.36	0.67	8.00	5.05	0.22	6.45	—	45.00
173	OLIVE, DRIED	,,	,,	—	30.07	5.24	51.90	10.45	2.34	27.02	2.52	2.50	0.06	0.30	0.46	0.36	0.22	0.06	—	33.50
174	SUNFLOWER SEED	SR	,,	—	10.50	14.20	32.30	14.50	3.50	6.12	2.80	2.87	4.65	0.60	13.38	0.87	5.54	0.90	—	37.73
175	SESAME	,,	,,	—	9.14	35.99	24.62	22.83	7.42	—	—	—	—	—	—	—	—	—	—	—
	GROUP D																			
176	COTTAGE CHEESE	SAR	,,	192	72.55	20.90	1.00	4.30	1.25	5.40	0.90	14.35	1.00	0.30	15.35	0.60	—	7.10	—	45.00
177	CREAM	,,	,,	245	74.00	2.50	18.50	4.50	0.50	5.15	1.55	4.25	0.60	0.50	3.90	0.45	—	2.00	—	18.40
178	BUTTER, COW'S	,,	,,	752	11.00	1.00	85.00	—	3.00	1.75	12.10	0.90	0.18	0.05	0.12	6.85	—	11.75	—	33.70
179	EGG, WHOLE	,,	,,	171	73.70	12.55	12.10	0.55	1.10	6.27	9.56	4.56	0.46	0.17	15.72	0.13	0.13	3.72	—	40.22
180	EGG, WHITE	,,	,,	50	85.75	12.70	0.25	0.70	0.60	13.21	13.30	1.18	1.18	0.25	1.85	0.88	0.45	12.08	—	44.38
181	EGG, YOLK	,,	,,	381	50.65	16.20	31.95	0.10	1.10	2.70	1.44	3.17	0.51	0.40	15.22	—	0.21	0.45	—	24.10

ABBREVIATIONS: C=Cosmic S=Solar T=Terrestrial H=Human A=Animal R=Radiations

REFERENCE No.	NAMES OF FOODS (Continued)	IMPONDERABLE COSMOVITAL FORCES			AVERAGE CHEMICAL COMPOSITION PER CENT					COMPOSITION OF MINERAL MATTER IN 1000 PARTS OF WATER FREE SUBSTANCE										
										ACID BINDING ELEMENTS					ACID FORMING ELEMENTS					
		PREDOMINANT RADIATIONS	PREDOMINANT VITAMINS	CALORIES Per 100 Grams	WATER	PROTEIN	FAT	CARBOHYDRATES (SUGAR, STARCH)	MINERAL MATTER	POTASSIUM K_2O	SODIUM Na_2O	CALCIUM CaO	MAGNESIUM MgO	IRON Fe_2O_3	PHOSPHORUS P_2O_5	SULPHUR SO_3	SILICON SiO_2	CHLORINE	FLUORINE	TOTAL
	CATEGORY V	SR	B		35, 15 and 10% OF THE DAILY RATION — COOKED VEGETABLES — CONSTRUCTIVE FOODS *(Permissible once or twice a week but not recommended)*															
	GROUP A (35%)																			
	All Vegetables of Category II in cooked form, and the following:—																			
182	PUMPKIN	..	..	25	91.47	1.10	0.13	6.50	0.70	13.85	15.22	5.55	2.45	1.88	23.80	1.73	5.27	0.30	—	70.05
183	LIMA BEAN, GREEN	..	..	32	68.50	7.10	0.70	22.00	1.70	33.90	4.75	1.40	3.60	0.14	6.60	3.10	—	0.50	—	53.99
184	KIDNEY BEAN, GREEN	..	..	132	86.90	3.90	0.20	8.30	0.70	23.30	1.70	2.75	1.65	0.05	5.65	7.00	—	1.90	—	44.00
185	STRING BEAN, FRESH	..	..	40	86.40	3.90	0.20	8.30	1.20	32.00	1.75	7.50	6.25	0.05	6.50	12.75	—	7.10	—	73.80
186	PEAS, GREEN	..	..	90	74.60	7.00	0.50	16.90	1.00	15.40	1.10	1.60	2.80	0.04	11.20	6.00	—	1.40	—	39.54
	GROUP B (15%)																			
187	EGG-PLANT	..	..	28	92.90	1.20	0.30	5.10	0.50	39.05	2.80	3.05	4.20	0.25	9.50	4.45	—	6.70	—	70.00
188	SOYA BEAN	..	..	442	10.75	34.00	16.80	33.70	4.75	24.65	0.60	3.45	3.45	0.28	17.50	2.65	0.27	0.40	—	53.25
189	LENTIL	..	..	337	16.06	25.70	1.90	53.30	3.04	11.60	4.60	2.10	0.90	0.60	12.20	1.20	—	1.50	—	34.70
190	MUSHROOM	TR	..	28	90.30	2.60	0.30	6.10	0.70	32.68	1.05	0.65	2.18	1.02	21.60	2.50	0.65	0.57	—	62.90
191	CHAMPIGNON	..	..	39	92.11	3.74	0.15	3.50	0.50	37.87	1.27	0.55	0.37	0.85	11.50	18.15	1.05	3.45	—	75.06
192	TRUFFLE	..	..	93	83.28	7.70	0.50	6.60	1.92	31.50	1.50	8.15	1.05	4.65	27.65	5.00	0.20	1.10	—	80.80
	GROUP C (10%)																			
193	BEAN, DRIED	SR	..	332	21.84	24.30	1.60	49.00	3.26	15.85	0.42	1.91	2.73	0.19	14.86	1.30	0.25	0.69	—	38.20
194	BEAN, BLACKEYE	..	..	338	11.23	21.43	1.28	61 28	4.78	—	—	—	—	—	—	—	—	—	—	—
195	HORSE-BEAN	..	..	342	28.25	18.00	0.50	50.50	2.75	15.25	0.40	0.15	0.30	0.10	14.30	1.15	—	0.60	—	32.25
196	LIMA BEAN, DRIED	..	..	—	10.40	18.10	1.50	65.90	4.10	27.60	4 10	1.25	3.10	0.01	6.10	2.60	—	0.04	—	44.80
197	KIDNEY BEAN, DRIED	..	..	334	17.44	23.12	2.28	53.63	3.53	18.00	0.58	2.60	3.00	0.13	14.30	1.65	0.23	0.34	—	40.83
198	PEAS, DRIED	..	..	336	20.37	22.85	1.80	52.40	2.58	13.06	0.30	1.45	2.42	0.24	10.87	1.03	1.27	0.53	—	31.17
199	COW PEAS, DRIED	..	..	348	13.00	21.40	1.40	60.80	3.40	21.00	2.40	1.50	3.15	—	6.85	3.60	—	0.60	—	39.10
200	CHICK PEAS (GARBANZAS)	..	..	323	30.24	13.00	1.60	51.50	3.76	8.10	0.40	1.45	18.35	0.80	13.10	1.10	—	0.95	—	44.25

ABBREVIATIONS: C=Cosmic S=Solar T=Terrestrial H=Human A=Animal R=Radiations

APPENDIX

VARIOUS TABLES AND CHARTS

TABLE OF FRUITS AND VEGETABLES WITH THE CHIEF CURATIVE MEDICINES CONTAINED IN THEM

Apples	SODA, Phosphorus
Asparagus	Saltpetre
Barley	PHOSPHORUS, IRON, POTASSIUM, magnesia, lime
Bread (wholemeal)	PHOSPHORUS, IRON, magnesia, potassium, lime
Cabbage	ARSENIC, SULPHUR, iodine, phosphorus, soda
Carrots	SODA, IRON
Celery	AROMATICS, SALTPETRE
Cereals (whole)	LIME, MAGNESIA, iron, phosphorus, soda
Chervil	Aromatics
Chives	AROMATICS, silica
Cress	IODINE, SULPHUR
Dahlia (rhizome)	INULIN
Garlic	ALLYL, SULPHUR, IODINE, silica, aromatics
Jerusalem Artichoke	INULIN, SALTPETRE
Leeks	IRON, MAGNESIA, SILICA, SODA, sulphur, saltpetre
Lettuce	LACTUCARIUM, iron, magnesia
Oats	SODA, IRON, phoshorus, magnesia, lime.
Onions	SULPHUR, SILICA, iodine, iron, saltpetre, aromatics
Parsley	AROMATICS
Plums	Iron, phosphorus
Radishes	IODINE, SULPHUR
Raspberries	SALICIN, lime, iron
Shallot	AROMATICS, silica
Spinach	SODA, IRON, lime
Spring Onions	AROMATICS, SILICA
Strawberries	SALICIN, lime, iron;
Thyme	THYMOL, AROMATICS
Tomatoes	Iron, phosphorus
Turnips	ARSENIC, magnesia, saltpetre
Wheat	PHOSPHORUS, magnesia, lime, soda, iron

FOODS STRENGTHENING BONES, BLOOD AND NERVES

(Arranged according to the amount of three specific elements, *iron, lime and phosphorus*, contained in each, compared with an equal weight of milk, which is taken as the standard food with coefficient 1.)

BLOOD TONICS (IRON)
(Quantity per 1000 grammes)

Lettuce	18	Wheat	5	Raspberry	2
Barley	18	Wholemeal Bread	5	Carrot	2
Oats	9	Cabbage	5	Tomato	2
Onion	7½	Plum	2	Egg	2
Leek	5	Strawberry	2	Milk	1

BONE AND GENERAL CONDITION TONICS (LIME)
(Quantity per 1000 grammes)

Cabbage	2	Egg	1	Wheat	½
Cauliflower	2	Milk	1	Wholemeal Bread	½
Strawberry	2	Carrot	¾	Onion	¼
Raspberry	2	Barley	½	Tomato	¼
Oats	1¼				

NERVE TONICS (Phosphorus)

(Quantity per 1000 grammes)

Barley	10	Cabbage	2¼	Potato	1
Wheat	10	Milk	1	Plum	1
Oats	9½	Onion	1	Strawberry	1
Wholemeal Bread	8	Lettuce	1	Raspberry	1
Egg	4½	Carrot	1	Tomato	1

DETERGENT FOODS

Foods which cleanse the alimentary canal and large intestine and alkalise excessive acidity of the stomach and blood, arranged in order of their alkaline (potassium or soda) salt content. Those with a large amount of alkalines are particularly suitable foods for patients suffering from stomach troubles (acidity, heartburn, hyperchloridria, arthritis, constipation, or enteritis.)

(Quantity of salt of potassium per 1000 grammes)

Barley	9½	Lettuce	3¾	Spinach	2½
Potato	6½	Leek	3¾	Onion	1¾
Oats	5½	Apple	3¾	Egg	1¾
Wheat	4¾	Cabbage	3¾	Milk	1
Wholemeal Bread	4¾	Carrot	3		

(Quantity of salt of soda per 1000 grammes)

Spinach	21	Carrot	4¾	Wholemeal Bread	1½
Egg	6¾	Barley	3¾	Milk	1
Cabbage	5¾	Lettuce	2½	Potato	¾
Leek	5¾	Oats	1½	Onion	¾
Apple	5¾	Wheat	1½		

TABLE OF MEDICINAL PROPERTIES WITH THE FRUITS AND VEGETABLES CONTAINING THEM

Property	*Where Found*	*Remarks*
Allyl	Garlic	Accelerates circulation of the blood. Varicose veins, arteriosclerosis, difficult periods (dysmenorrhea), change of life (menopause). Antiseptic. Good for those who feel the cold on account of its intense stimulation. Aids digestion. (*Vide* Apiol.)
Antiseptics	All fresh vegetables, especially aromatic herbs and watery, acid fruits	These are natural antiseptics and most effective in their raw state. Should be included in the diet of patients with all kinds of enteritis as it is always due to putrefaction of undigested flesh foods in the stomach, and their subsequent decomposition in the ileo-caecal fossa.

Property	*Where Found*	*Remarks*
Apiol	Parsley	Apiol, the active principle in parsley is one of the best things for stimulating blood circulation. It also aids digestion. The stomach, like the rest of the digestive organs, expends a good deal of energy supplied by the nervous system. Nervous activity increases with acceleration of the blood round the nervous fibrils. (*Vide* "Allyl" for other uses of Apiol.)
Aromatics	Celery, chervil, chives, garlic, onion, parsley, shallot, thyme	Aromatics stimulate the appetite and aid digestion. They are antiseptic (the genuine intestinal antiseptics) and consequently blood-cleansers. They should be taken by sufferers from arthritis, rheumatism, phlebitis, varicose veins, bronchitis and all skin diseases.
Arsenic	Cabbage, turnip	The human body contains a few milligrammes of arsenic, which is a strength-giving metalloid. (Greek 'arsen,'—strong and 'nikan,'=to conquer). It is therefore a necessary element in consumptive conditions *e.g.* tuberculosis.
Bitters	Chicory (all kinds including endive), Dandelion	Bitters are stomachics and blood-cleansers, so they should be taken for anæmia, loss of appetite, impurity of the blood, etc.
Camphor	Bay-tree	Camphor is extracted from the camphor tree, a kind of bay tree. It is a very valuable antiseptic, being of vegetable origin. The bay tree itself also contains some camphor. Its use in the kitchen is recommended for keeping the alimentary canal in good condition.
Diuretics	Culinary roots, green vegetables & watery fruits	These are natural diuretics for the obvious reason that on an average they contain 90 per cent of vegetable water (their blood), and water is the best of diuretics. Good as blood purifiers, for relieving inflammation of the digestive organs, and for congestion.
Inulin	Salsify, Jerusalem artichoke, dahlia rhizome	Inulin is invert sugar, without the intervention of the pancreatic juices. Consequently it is suitable for diabetics.

Property	*Where Found*	*Remarks*
Iodine	**Cabbage, cress, garlic, onion, radish**	**Iodine relieves congestion of the lymphatic ganglia and aids phagocytosis in the body's defensive system. At the same time it stimulates glandular secretion, thus increasing the rate of change of the cells. It is an antiscorbutic and relieves congestion. Good for rickets, lymphatism, scrofula, bronchitis, obesity, tuberculosis, skin diseases.**
Iron	**Barley, kohlrabi, leek, lettuce, oats, onion, spinach**	**Iron regenerates and strengthens the red blood corpuscles. (Anæmia, chlorosis, debility, growing age, tuberculosis.)**
Lactucarium	**Cos lettuce, lettuce**	**Lactucarium has the same calming, soporific properties as opium. These vegetables are good, therefore, for people suffering from insomnia, nervous internal inflammation such as bronchitis, etc.**
Laxatives	**Bitter vegetables, watery fruits**	**These are both excellent laxatives. Fruit should be taken alone and in considerable quantity to get the best results.**
Lime	**Cabbage, raspberry, spinach, strawberry, whole cereals, drinking water**	**Lime strengthens the bones by furnishing them with their chief component. (Rickets, general debility.) It also calcifies abscesses. (Abscesses, furunculosis, tuberculosis.)**
Magnesia	**Apple, carrot, celery, leek, lettuce, radish, turnip, watery fruits, whole cereals, wholemeal wheat bread**	**Magnesia regenerates the fibrous substance of the nerves, and in conjunction with phosphorus is suitable for rebuilding weakened nerves. It is particularly valuable in neuritis, polyneuritis and general diseases such as debility, tuberculosis, diabetes, cancer, etc.**
Mucilages	**Corn salad, garlic, leek, onion, purslane, apple, lemon, orange, and all other watery fruits**	**Mucilage is of the greatest importance in aiding the lubricating mucus of our bodies which is in the joints (synovia), intestines and bronchial tubes. It is good for people with over-stiff joints, for sufferers from constipation, as lubrication of the intestines promotes defecation, and bronchitis where it makes the bronchioles slide upon one another more easily and helps to get rid of their phlegm.**

Property	*Where Found*	*Remarks*
Phosphorus	Barley, egg, oats, wheat, wholemeal wheat bread	Phosphorus regenerates nervous energy. Egg should be used where quick results are wanted as its yolk contains phosphorated fat (lecithin) assimilable in its ideal form. For lasting effects cereals are preferable. General application—in neurosis, nervous diseases, debility, growing age, tuberculosis.
Potassium (Salts of)	Barley, lentils, oats, potato, wheat, wholemeal wheat bread	Salts of potassium are detergents (cleansers) of the alimentary canal and large intestine. They also alkalinise excessive acidity of the stomach and blood.
Salicin	Raspberry, strawberry	Real salicin extracted from meadow-sweet (ulmaria) is the ideal specific for gout, rheumatism, gravel and for alleviation of gravel pains. Fruits with salicin in them should be taken by sufferers from these complaints, even though their consumption is attended by nettle-rash. This is a proof of the salicin's having thrown out the toxins causing trouble.
Saltpetre	Asparagus, carrot, Chinese artichoke, Jerusalem artichoke, garlic, leek, onion, potato, turnip, yam	The natural salts of nitre, which ordinary roots contain, are excellent diuretics, helping to purify the blood by causing profuse urination, and by passing into the blood, to ease inflammation of the liver, kidneys, prostate and bladder. (Asparagus not to be used in nephritis or cystitis.) They are also good for arthritis, rheumatism (other than asparagus, as it contains oxalates), phlebitis, congested organs and skin disease.
Silica	Chive, garlic, leek, onion, shallot	Silica combined with lime strengthens and keeps supple bones and arteries. It also plays a part in the formation of skin, of the membranes of our viscera, of the nails and the hair on our heads and bodies. It is therefore appropriate in rickets and arterio-sclerosis and to strengthen our intestinal organs, accelerate the cure of skin diseases, make the nails strong and flexible, and make the hair grow again (in this case used in conjunction with sulphur).
Soda (Salts of)	Apple, cabbage, carrot, leek, lentil, spinach	Salts of soda, like salts of potassium, are detergents (cleansers) of the alimentary canal and large intestine. They also alkalinise excessive acidity of the stomach and blood. They are milder in action than potassium.

Property	*Where Found*	*Remarks*
Sulphur	Cabbage, cress, egg (chiefly the white), garlic, leek, onion, radish	Sulphur is an antiseptic which spreads to every part of the body as a sulphurous gas. It is therefore one of the most active blood purifiers. It may be used with great success in its edible form in intestinal infections, skin diseases, bronchial diseases, rheumatism and alopecia (loss of hair) due to an infection of the pilary glands.
Thymol	Thyme	The thymol and camphor extracted from thyme is a powerful antiseptic for the intestinal tracts, the blood and the bronchiæ. It is a most excellent vermifuge and tænicide.

VITAMINOTHERAPEUTIC MEDICINES

Fire and Life

Every living creature other than man eats things in their raw, uncooked state. Fire transforms or destroys everything it touches. Of a living food adapted to the purpose of nutrition and assimilation it makes a dead food that is unsuitable for maintaining health and life. The same is true of natural drinks.

Animals show that this is so. While they live in their natural conditions they are free from disease, but they lose their health as soon as they come to live with human beings and are fed with cooked foods.

Crudities as Medicines

Below we give two tables of vitaminotherapeutic medicines: correct diet makes every other medicine unnecessary.

IMPORTANT ELEMENTS

The most important elements are contained in organic state in the following foods:

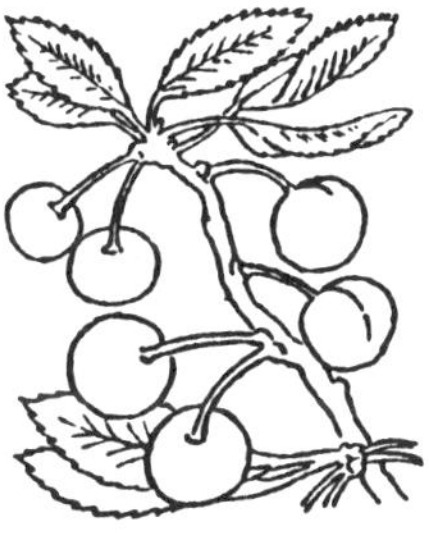

TABLE No. 1

Calcium in	*Iron in*	*Magnesium in*	*Phosphorus in*
Asparagus	Asparagus	Almond	Apple
Cabbage	Barley	Barley	Cauliflower
Cheese (fresh)	Carrot	Coconut	Cucumber
Dandelion	Kohlrabi	Dandelion	Cumin
Egg (yolk)	Lettuce	Maize	Egg (yolk)
Grape	Onion	Oats	Fennel
Kohlrabi	Prune	Orange	Milk
Leek	Radish	Rye	Nuts
Lettuce	Redcurrant	Wheat	Roots
Nettle	Spinach		Wheat
Onion	Strawberry		
Orange			
Prune			
Radish			
Redcurrant			
Salsify			
Spinach			
Strawberry			
Strawberry leaves			

Potassium in	*Silicium in*	*Sodium in*	*Sulphur in*
Balm	Asparagus	Apple	Cabbage (white-heart)
Cabbage	Barley	Asparagus (young)	Cauliflower
Camomile	Dandelion root	Cabbage	Kohlrabi
Centaury	Oats	Carrot	Leek
Dandelion	Potato	Cucumber	Lettuce
Grape	Salsify	Dandelion	
Kohlrabi	Strawberry	Fennel	
Lettuce	Vegetables	Lettuce	
Olive	Wheat	Milk	
Potato		Radish	
Prune		Sorrel	
Rhubarb		Spinach	
		Strawberry	

TABLE No. II

CONTENTS OF 100 GRAMMES OF FRUIT

	Albumen	*Fat*	*Carbo-hydrates*	*Cellulose*	*Ash*	*Water*	*Calories*
Apple .	0.06	—	14	2	0.4	84	59
Apricot .	0.15	—	12	—	0.7	85	53
Banana .	0.2	—	23	0.8	0.9	74	98
Cherry .	0.1	—	16	1.5	0.5	82	69
Fig (dried).	0.5	3.5	61	7	2.5	26	262
Grape .	0.1	—	18	1.2	0.5	79	76
Pear. ..	0.06	—	14	3.5	0.4	84	59
Plum .	0.1	—	17	—	0.1	81	73
Raspberry.	0.2	—	8	5.7	0.6	84	37
Strawberry	0.2	—	9	3	0.7	85	41
Chestnut .	1	4.1	40	1.6	1.4	47	227
Hazel-nut .	2.8	63	7	6	2.5	7	684
Walnut .	0.7	58	3	3	1.7	1.7	663

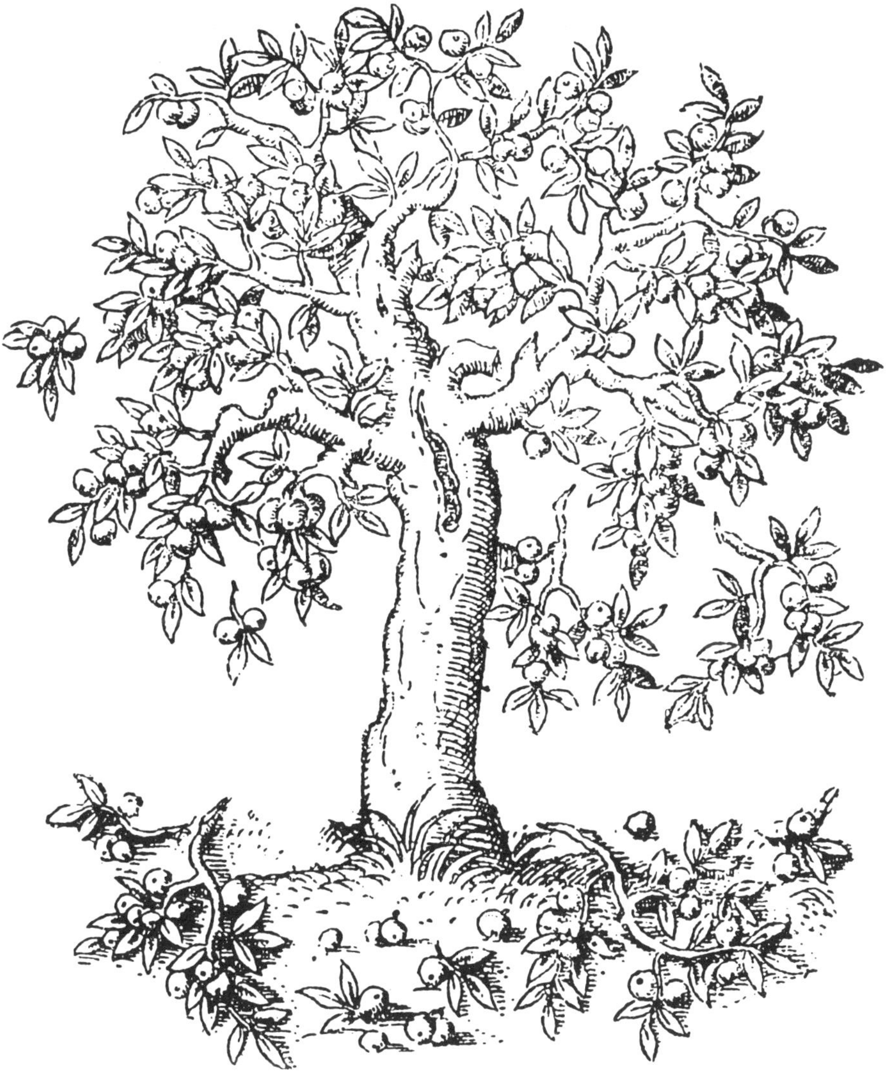

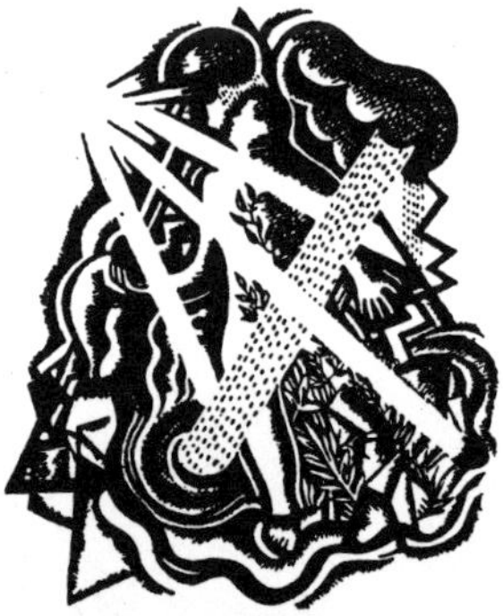

The Twelve Preconditions
of an Individual's Degree of Perfection

(from the original *Cosmos, Man and Society*, by the author)

Individual and bodily perfection, health and well-being, necessarily depend on the degree of evolution reached by the twelve known and less-well known senses. This is directly dependent upon the following factors in physical, mental and moral health.

1. Power of accumulating the energy of the eternal cosmic ocean of the higher cosmic radiations.
2. Capacity of power of breathing.
3. Generation of electrical fluid by the expansion of the ganglia of the nervous system.
4. Regularization of the blood circulation in the body by perfect functioning of the lungs.
5. Rhythmic distribution of the blood in the body by the movement of the heart.
6. Equal development of all the cells of the brain.
7. Awakening of the power of thought by the vibrations of the spinal cord.
8. Expansion of the magnetic circuits by the vibrations of the senses of the sympathetic nervous system.
9. Perfect assimilation of food after complete digestion.
10. Purification of the body by its appropriate organs.
11. Generation of vital fluid or regeneration by the organs charged with the conservation of life.
12. Economy in every energy and consciousness of all in existence (optimal and omnilateral orientation).

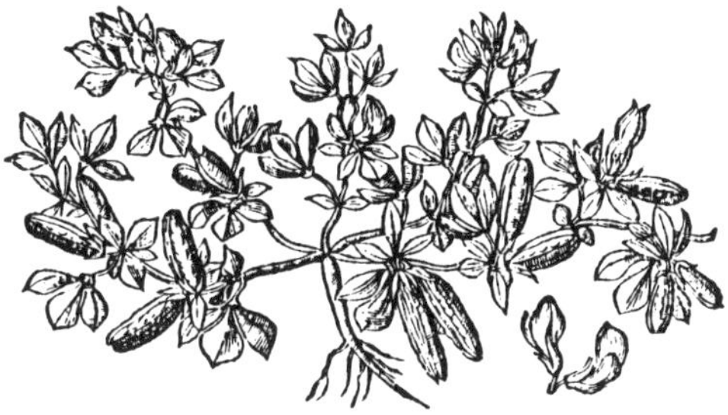

EPILOGUE

THE GOLDEN RULES OF HEALTH AND HAPPINESS

Spend as much time as possible in fresh, pure air.

Always take a cold or lukewarm shower in the morning when you awaken, and in the evening before you go to bed.

Devote one half-day a week to alternate sunbaths and waterbaths, swimming where possible. (The early-morning sun is best, in moderation, to avoid harmful ultra-violet rays.)

Take a walk after lunch and dinner every day for 30 or 40 minutes, breathing fresh air deeply and rhythmically.

Do some simple physical culture exercises for 10 or 15 minutes every morning on rising.

Always sleep in a cool, airy and quiet place.

Follow the middle path of moderation and naturalness in all things, particularly in food, rest, work, recreation, and sleep.

Beware of psychological toxins (inharmonious thoughts and feelings) even more than chemical poisons. Be an optimist and have confidence in yourself, in human progress, and in the healing forces of nature.

Be a sincere altruist and love and help others. Appreciate people's good qualities and forgive their bad ones.

Enjoy the beauties of nature and the masterpieces of literature, the arts, and philosophy. Fill your life with the great music of masters such as Beethoven, Bach and Mozart.

Study and observe the natural and cosmic laws, and live in complete harmony with the natural and cosmic forces.

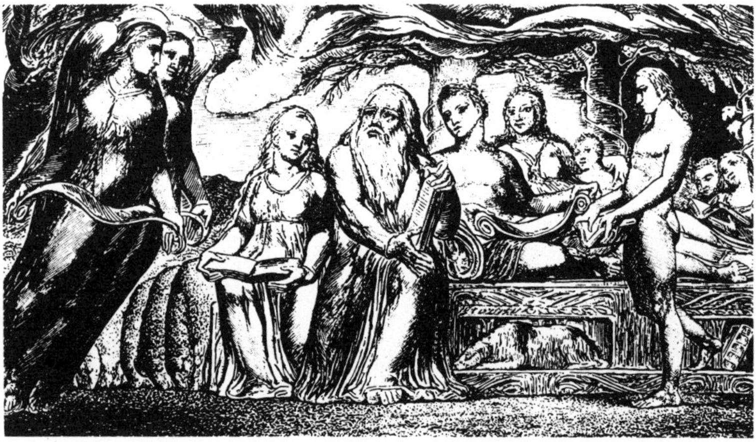

THE STORY OF THE ESSENE GOSPEL OF PEACE

Translated by Edmond Bordeaux Szekely

In Four Volumes

It was in 1928 that Edmond Bordeaux Szekely first published his translation of Book One of *The Essene Gospel of Peace,* an ancient manuscript he had found in the Secret Archives of the Vatican as the result of limitless patience, faultless scholarship, and unerring intuition. This story is told in his book, *The Discovery of the Essene Gospel of Peace,* published in 1975. The English version of Book One appeared in 1937, and ever since, the little volume has traveled over the world, appearing in many different languages, gaining every year more and more readers, until now, still with no commercial advertisement, over a million copies have been sold in the United States alone. It was not until almost fifty years after the first French translation that Book Two and Book Three appeared *(The Unknown Books of the Essenes* and *Lost Scrolls of the Essene Brotherhood),* achieving rapidly the popularity of Book One.

In 1981, Book Four, *The Teachings of the Elect,* was published posthumously according to Dr. Szekely's wishes, representing yet another fragment of the complete manuscript which exists in Aramaic in the Secret Archives of the Vatican and in old Slavonic in the Royal Library of the Habsburgs (now the property of the Austrian government). The poetic style of the translator brings to vivid reality the exquisitely beautiful words of Jesus and the Elders of the Essene Brotherhood. Some of the chapters: The Essene Communions. The Sevenfold Peace. The Holy Streams of Life, Light, and Sound. The Gift of the Humble Grass.

All four volumes of *The Essene Gospel of Peace* are available in English from the International Biogenic Society mailing address: I.B.S. Internacional, Box 849, Nelson, B.C., Canada V1L 6A5. A free descriptive catalogue of these and all the collected works of Edmond Bordeaux Szekely will be gladly sent upon request.

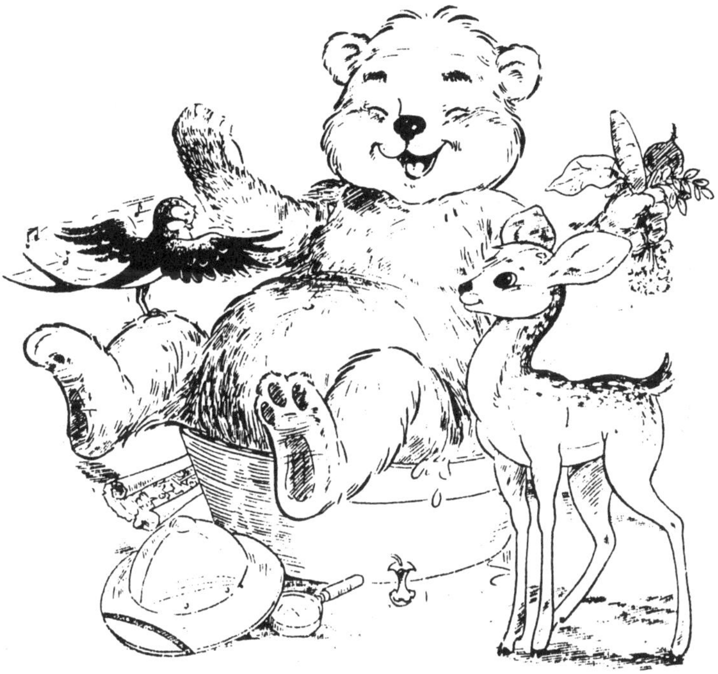

. . . from the Essene Gospel of Peace. . .

". . . but he who kills a beast without a cause, though the beast attack him not, through lust for slaughter, or for its flesh, or for its hide, or yet for its tusks, evil is the deed which he does, for he is turned into a wild beast himself. Wherefore is his end also as the end of the wild beasts."

"Kill neither man, nor beasts, nor yet the food which goes into your mouth. For if you eat living food, the same will quicken you, but if you kill your food, the dead food will kill you also. For life comes only from life, and from death comes always death. . ."

"Behold, I have given you every herb-bearing seed, which is upon the face of all the earth, and every tree, in the which is the fruit of a tree yielding seed; to you it shall be for meat. But flesh, and the blood which quickens it, shall ye not eat."

"For I tell you truly, he who kills, kills himself, and whoso eats the flesh of slain beasts, eats of the body of death."

–The Essene Gospel of Peace, Book One
translated by Edmond Bordeaux Szekely

THE ESSENE WAY
BIOGENIC LIVING

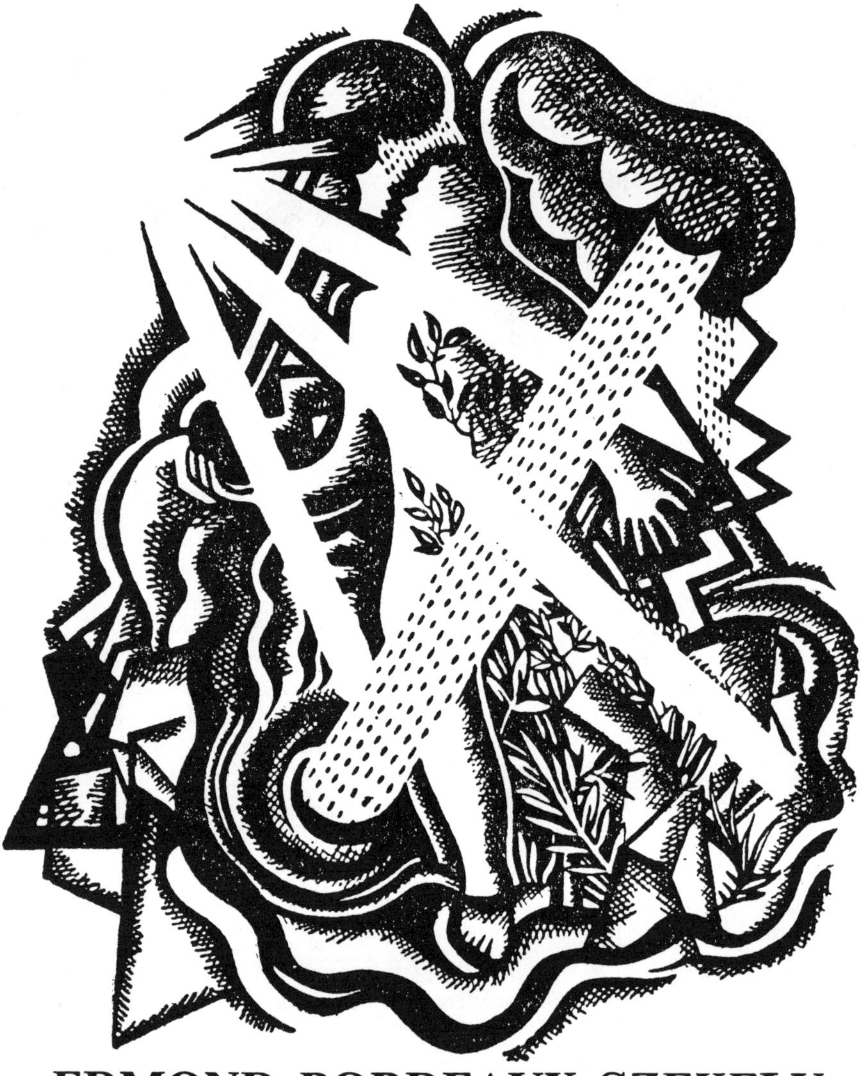

EDMOND BORDEAUX SZEKELY

The Textbook of the International Biogenic Society

Soft-Cover Edition (sent free to all new members of the I.B.S.) U.S. $8.80
Case-Bound Edition U.S. $15.00

Add 15% for postage & handling and send orders to our mailing address:
International Biogenic Society, P.O. Box 849, Nelson, B.C., Canada V1L 6A5
Please remember to send checks in U.S. funds only.

APPLICATION FOR ASSOCIATE MEMBERSHIP
INTERNATIONAL BIOGENIC SOCIETY

Please return to: *I.B.S. Internacional*
Box 849, Nelson, B.C.
Canada V1L 6A5

*Name*______________________________

*Address*______________________________

*City*____________*State/Prov.*__________*Zip/Code*_______

*Age*___*Profession*______________________________

*Previous Experience*______________________________

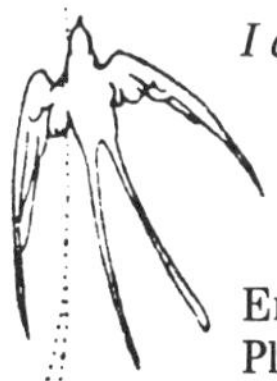

I am interested in:

____*becoming an Associate Member of the I.B.S.*

____*becoming a Teacher of Biogenic Living.*

Enclosed is my annual Associate Membership fee of $20.00. Please mail my membership card, your next issue of the Periodical Review, *The Essene Way*, and my copy of *The Essene Way—Biogenic Living*, my most important textbook and encyclopedia of ancient wisdom and modern practice. I understand I will receive a 20% discount on all publications as an Associate Member, but only if I order *directly* from I.B.S. Internacional.

Please make your check in U.S. currency out to
I.B.S. INTERNACIONAL.

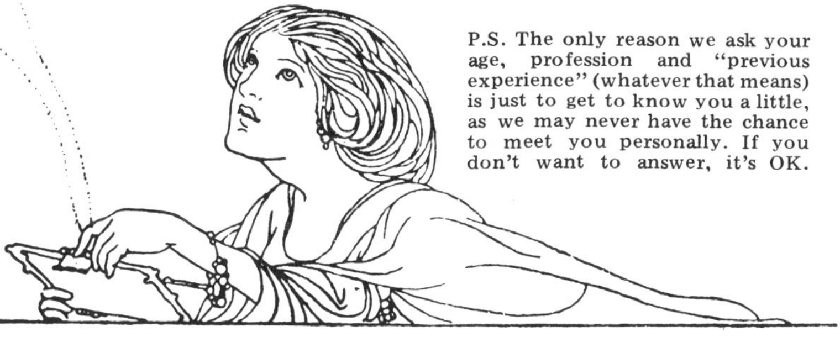

P.S. The only reason we ask your age, profession and "previous experience" (whatever that means) is just to get to know you a little, as we may never have the chance to meet you personally. If you don't want to answer, it's OK.

RECOMMENDED BOOKS FOR STUDY

Many members who have not yet started study groups or live far from book stores and/or like-minded individuals, are interested in a systematic program of home study. The following books are recommended for such a program, and provide an excellent foundation for study of *The Essene Way of Biogenic Living*, especially when coordinated with the methods outlined in *The Art of Study: the Sorbonne Method.*

Please send me the following books:

____*The Essene Gospel of Peace, Book One $1.00*
____*The Essene Gospel of Peace, Book Two $7.50*
____*The Essene Gospel of Peace, Book Three $7.50*
____*The Essene Gospel of Peace, Book Four $5.95*
____*The Essene Way-Biogenic Living $8.80 (free with membership)*
____*The Biogenic Revolution $9.50*
____*The Chemistry of Youth $7.50*
____*From Enoch to the Dead Sea Scrolls $5.95*
____*The Essene Book of Creation $4.50*
____*The Essene Code of Life $3.50*
____*The Essene Science of Life $3.50*
____*Essene Communions with the Infinite $4.50*
____*Discovery of the Essene Gospel of Peace $5.95*
____*The Essene Book of Asha $7.50*
____*Books, Our Eternal Companions $3.50*
____*Cosmos, Man and Society $6.80*
____*Search for the Ageless, Volume One $7.80*
____*Search for the Ageless, Volume Two $8.80*
____*The Ecological Health Garden, the Book of Survival $5.95*
____*The Art of Study: the Sorbonne Method $3.50*

______*Total*
______*Add 15% for Postage & Handling ($2.00 minimum)*

*U.S. $*____________*Total Amount Enclosed*

Please address all orders and correspondence to:

I.B.S. INTERNACIONAL
Box 849, Nelson, B.C., Canada V1L 6A5

*Name*______________________________

*Address*______________________________

*City, State/Province, Zip/Code*____________________

All orders must be pre-paid. Minimum order: $5.00, minimum postage and handling: $1.50. Please make check, draft or money order in *U.S. currency, drawn on a U.S. bank*, out to I.B.S. Internacional. Please allow 4 weeks for processing, more for foreign orders. Members of the I.B.S. may deduct 20% and *active* Teachers of Biogenic Living may deduct 40% (both must have valid membership cards for the current year). Dealers and distributors, please write to above address for discount infomation. *All sales are considered final.*